DIALYSIS DIET MEAL PLANS

Healthy and Delicious Kidney-Friendly Recipes for Every Meal

Dr Lily Morgan

COPYRIGHT PAGE

All rights reserved. The copyright holder must provide written permission before any part of this publication can be republished in any manner, such as photocopying, scanning, or other methods.

Copyright ©2023

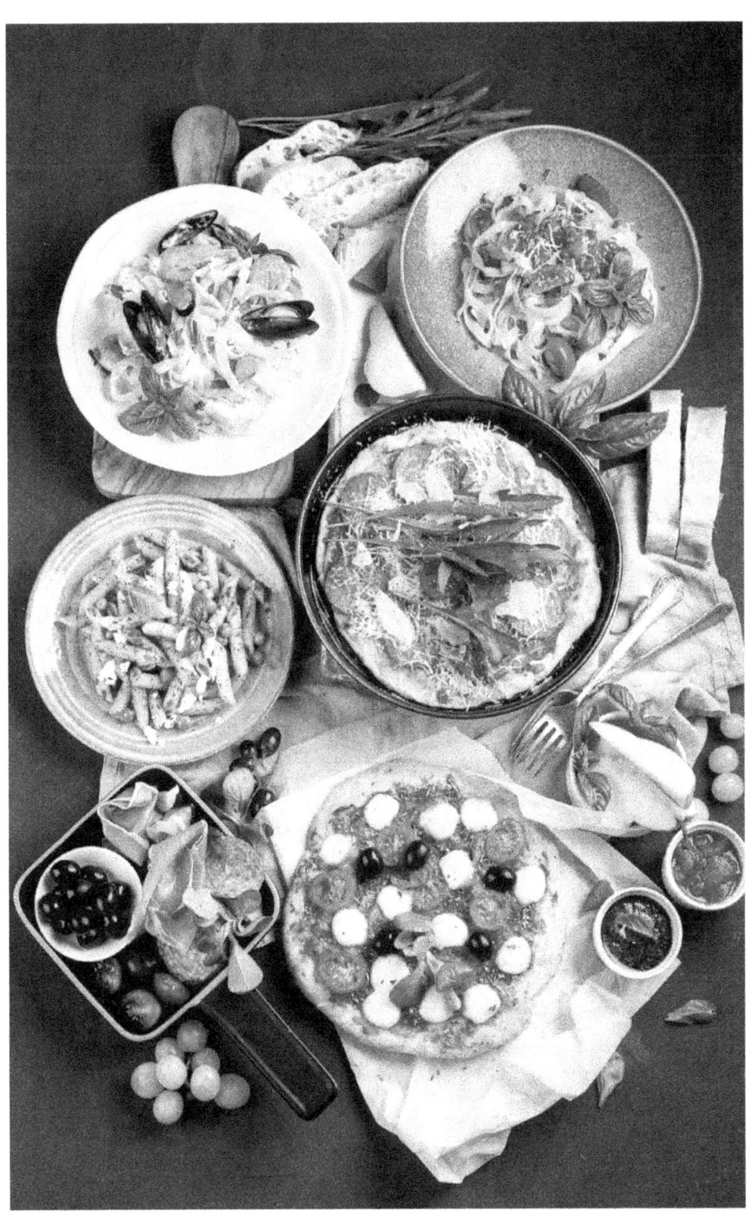

TABLE OF CONTENTS

Chapter 3: Lunch Recipes 37

INTRODUCTION

When facing the challenges of dialysis, one aspect that often takes center stage in your healthcare journey is nutrition. The dialysis diet is not just a mere list of restrictions; it's a crucial component of your well-being. Understanding the intricate relationship between the dialysis diet and your overall health is essential for a balanced and fulfilling life while on this path. In this article, we'll delve into the complexities of this diet and explore the profound significance of nutrition in dialysis.

The Dialysis Diet Unveiled:

The dialysis diet is carefully designed to manage specific aspects of your health, particularly when your kidneys are unable to perform their natural filtration functions. It's a well-thought-out plan that primarily focuses on controlling the intake of key nutrients, such as sodium, potassium, and phosphorus. By regulating these elements, the diet aims to prevent complications and maintain an optimal balance in your body.

Sodium: The Silent Culprit

One of the key players in the dialysis diet is sodium. While it often gets a bad rap, sodium control is pivotal. Excessive sodium intake can lead to fluid retention and high blood pressure, which are common challenges for individuals on dialysis. Therefore, the diet emphasizes limiting sodium, making it essential to read food labels and choose fresh, unprocessed ingredients whenever possible.

Potassium: Balancing Act

Potassium plays a vital role in muscle and nerve function. However, when your kidneys are compromised, maintaining the right potassium levels is crucial. High potassium levels can result in heart irregularities and muscle weakness. The dialysis diet helps control potassium intake by reducing foods rich in this mineral, such as bananas, oranges, and potatoes.

Phosphorus: The Stealthy Offender

Phosphorus is another mineral that needs careful monitoring. Excess phosphorus can lead to brittle bones and cardiovascular complications. Dialysis patients often need to restrict their phosphorus intake and take phosphate binders to prevent absorption in the gut.

Protein and Calories: The Balancing Act

Protein and calorie intake is an essential part of the dialysis diet. It's important to strike a balance between getting enough protein for tissue repair and maintaining a healthy weight. Registered dietitians work with dialysis patients to create meal plans that provide adequate protein and calories while considering individual needs.

The Role of Fluids

Fluid management is a fundamental aspect of the dialysis diet. Restricting fluids helps prevent fluid overload and high blood pressure. Dialysis patients must carefully monitor their fluid intake and make adjustments based on their treatment schedule.

Importance of Nutrition in Dialysis:

The importance of nutrition in the dialysis journey cannot be overstated. A well-managed diet can significantly impact your overall health and quality of life. Proper nutrition can help:

1. **Manage Symptoms**: A well-balanced diet can alleviate symptoms like fatigue, nausea, and muscle cramps that are often associated with dialysis.

2. **Support Vital Functions**: Proper nutrition is vital for supporting essential bodily functions, including tissue repair, immune system health, and energy production.

3. **Reduce Complications:** The dialysis diet is structured to minimize complications like fluid overload, high blood pressure, and mineral imbalances, which are common in dialysis patients.

4. **Improve Quality of Life:** With the right diet, you can enjoy a better quality of life, with improved energy levels and overall well-being.

Understanding the intricacies of the dialysis diet and recognizing the critical role of nutrition in dialysis is an empowering step in your journey towards better health. By working closely with healthcare professionals and embracing a diet tailored to your unique needs, you can navigate the challenges of dialysis with confidence and vitality. Remember, it's not just about restriction; it's about finding balance and living your best life, even in the face of adversity.

Chapter 1: 30-Day Meal Plan

Week 1:

Day 1:

- Breakfast: Creamy Oatmeal with Berries
- Lunch: Chicken and Vegetable Stir-Fry
- Dinner: Baked Salmon with Dill
- Snacks: Cucumber Slices with Hummus
- Dessert: Berry Sorbet

Day 2:

- Breakfast: Scrambled Egg Whites with Spinach
- Lunch: Tuna Salad with Avocado
- Dinner: Lemon Herb Grilled Chicken
- Snacks: Roasted Red Pepper Dip
- Dessert: Poached Pears

Day 3:

- Breakfast: Banana Nut Pancakes
- Lunch: Spinach and Feta Stuffed Chicken
- Dinner: Vegetable and Lentil Curry

- Snacks: Greek Salad Skewers
- Dessert: Applesauce with Cinnamon

Day 4:

- Breakfast: Greek Yogurt Parfait
- Lunch: Quinoa Salad with Roasted Vegetables
- Dinner: Beef and Vegetable Skewers
- Snacks: Mixed Nuts
- Dessert: Chia Seed Pudding

Day 5:

- Breakfast: Vegetable Omelette
- Lunch: Mediterranean Chicken Wrap
- Dinner: Spaghetti Squash with Pesto
- Snacks: Deviled Eggs
- Dessert: Angel Food Cake with Berries

Day 6:

- Breakfast: Apple Cinnamon Quinoa
- Lunch: Shrimp and Asparagus Salad
- Dinner: Tofu and Broccoli in Garlic Sauce
- Snacks: Guacamole with Veggie Sticks

- Dessert: Rice Pudding

Day 7:

- Breakfast: Smoothie Bowl
- Lunch: Turkey and Cranberry Sandwich
- Dinner: Roast Turkey with Gravy
- Snacks: Rice Cakes with Peanut Butter
- Dessert: Pumpkin Pie Smoothie

Week 2:

Day 8:

- Breakfast: Cottage Cheese and Fruit
- Lunch: Lentil Soup
- Dinner: Cod with Lemon Butter
- Snacks: Zucchini Fritters
- Dessert: Baked Apples

Day 9:

- Breakfast: Breakfast Muffins
- Lunch: Tofu and Broccoli Stir-Fry
- Dinner: Chickpea and Spinach Stew
- Snacks: Fruit Kabobs

- Dessert: Greek Yogurt with Honey

Day 10:

- Breakfast: Avocado Toast
- Lunch: Chicken Noodle Soup
- Dinner: Pork Tenderloin with Apples
- Snacks: Caprese Skewers
- Dessert: Chocolate Avocado Mousse

Day 11:

- Breakfast: Rice Pudding
- Lunch: Caprese Salad
- Dinner: Baked Eggplant Parmesan
- Snacks: Baked Sweet Potato Fries
- Dessert: Banana Ice Cream

Day 12:

- Breakfast: Breakfast Quesadilla
- Lunch: Salmon and Brown Rice
- Dinner: Salsa Chicken
- Snacks: Spinach and Artichoke Dip
- Dessert: Coconut Rice Pudding

Day 13:

- Breakfast: Breakfast Casserole
- Lunch: Egg Salad Lettuce Wraps
- Dinner: Teriyaki Beef Stir-Fry
- Snacks: Cottage Cheese with Pineapple
- Dessert: Fruit Salad

Day 14:

- Breakfast: Sweet Potato Hash
- Lunch: Black Bean and Corn Salad
- Dinner: Ratatouille
- Snacks: Edamame
- Dessert: Frozen Yogurt Bites

Week 3:

Day 15:

- Breakfast: Blueberry Waffles
- Lunch: Minestrone Soup
- Dinner: BBQ Pulled Chicken
- Snacks: Mini Quiches
- Dessert: Peach Cobbler

Day 16:

- Breakfast: Tofu Scramble
- Lunch: Hummus and Veggie Wrap
- Dinner: Shrimp Scampi
- Snacks: Baked Pita Chips with Salsa
- Dessert: Lemon Sorbet

Day 17:

- Breakfast: Pumpkin Spice Porridge
- Lunch: Stuffed Bell Peppers
- Dinner: Vegetable Lasagna
- Snacks: Tzatziki and Pita Bread
- Dessert: Carrot Cake Bites

Day 18:

- Breakfast: Chicken and Vegetable Stir-Fry
- Lunch: Tuna Salad with Avocado
- Dinner: Baked Salmon with Dill
- Snacks: Cucumber Slices with Hummus
- Dessert: Berry Sorbet

Day 19:

- Breakfast: Scrambled Egg Whites with Spinach
- Lunch: Spinach and Feta Stuffed Chicken
- Dinner: Lemon Herb Grilled Chicken
- Snacks: Roasted Red Pepper Dip
- Dessert: Poached Pears

Day 20:

- Breakfast: Banana Nut Pancakes
- Lunch: Quinoa Salad with Roasted Vegetables
- Dinner: Beef and Vegetable Skewers
- Snacks: Mixed Nuts
- Dessert: Chia Seed Pudding

Day 21:

- Breakfast: Greek Yogurt Parfait
- Lunch: Shrimp and Asparagus Salad
- Dinner: Tofu and Broccoli in Garlic Sauce
- Snacks: Deviled Eggs
- Dessert: Angel Food Cake with Berries

Week 4:

Day 22:

- Breakfast: Roast Turkey with Gravy
- Lunch: Chickpea and Spinach Stew
- Dinner: Pork Tenderloin with Apples
- Snacks: Caprese Skewers
- Dessert: Chocolate Avocado Mousse

Day 23:

- Breakfast: Cod with Lemon Butter
- Lunch: Baked Eggplant Parmesan
- Dinner: Salsa Chicken
- Snacks: Baked Sweet Potato Fries
- Dessert: Banana Ice Cream

Day 24:

- Breakfast: Chickpea and Spinach Stew
- Lunch: Caprese Salad
- Dinner: Baked Salmon with Dill
- Snacks: Zucchini Fritters
- Dessert: Fruit Salad

Day 25:

- Breakfast: Baked Eggplant Parmesan
- Lunch: Pork Tenderloin with Apples
- Dinner: BBQ Pulled Chicken
- Snacks: Fruit Kabobs
- Dessert: Greek Yogurt with Honey

Day 26:

- Breakfast: Salsa Chicken
- Lunch: Teriyaki Beef Stir-Fry
- Dinner: Vegetable Lasagna
- Snacks: Cottage Cheese with Pineapple
- Dessert: Coconut Rice Pudding

Day 27:

- Breakfast: BBQ Pulled Chicken
- Lunch: Shrimp Scampi
- Dinner: Beef and Rice Stuffed Peppers
- Snacks: Mini Quiches
- Dessert: Lemon Sorbet

Day 28:

- Breakfast: Vegetable Lasagna
- Lunch: Beef and Rice Stuffed Peppers
- Dinner: Ratatouille
- Snacks: Tzatziki and Pita Bread
- Dessert: Carrot Cake Bites

Day 29:

- Breakfast: Beef and Rice Stuffed Peppers
- Lunch: Teriyaki Beef Stir-Fry
- Dinner: Vegetable Lasagna
- Snacks: Tzatziki and Pita Bread
- Dessert: Carrot Cake Bites

Day 30:

- Breakfast: Vegetable Lasagna
- Lunch: Teriyaki Beef Stir-Fry
- Dinner: Vegetable Lasagna
- Snacks: Tzatziki and Pita Bread
- Dessert: Carrot Cake Bites

This concludes the 30-day meal plan with a variety of recipes. Remember to adjust portion sizes and ingredients to fit your specific dietary needs and preferences.

Chapter 2: Breakfast Recipes

In the realm of a balanced diet tailored for dialysis patients, breakfast becomes a significant foundation. The morning meal should not only be nutritious but also delicious. Let's explore a variety of hearty and wholesome breakfast recipes, each carefully crafted to fit your dietary needs.

Creamy Oatmeal with Berries

Ingredients:

- 1/2 cup rolled oats
- 1 cup low-sodium almond milk
- 1/4 cup fresh mixed berries
- 1 tablespoon honey (optional)

Instructions:

1. In a saucepan, combine oats and almond milk.
2. Cook over low heat, stirring occasionally, until the oats absorb the liquid and the mixture thickens.
3. Serve with a topping of fresh mixed berries and a drizzle of honey.

Scrambled Egg Whites with Spinach

Ingredients:

- 4 egg whites
- 1 cup fresh spinach leaves
- Salt and pepper to taste

Instructions:

1. Whisk egg whites in a bowl and season with salt and pepper.
2. In a non-stick skillet, lightly sauté the spinach until wilted.
3. Pour in the egg whites and scramble until cooked through.

Banana Nut Pancakes

Ingredients:

- 1 ripe banana, mashed
- 1/2 cup oat flour
- 1/4 cup chopped nuts
- 1/4 teaspoon cinnamon

Instructions:

1. Combine mashed banana, oat flour, chopped nuts, and cinnamon in a bowl.
2. Heat a non-stick pan and pour the batter to make pancakes. Cook until golden brown on both sides.

Greek Yogurt Parfait

Ingredients:

- 1/2 cup low-fat Greek yogurt
- 1/4 cup granola
- 1/4 cup mixed berries
- 1 tablespoon honey

Instructions:

1. In a glass, layer Greek yogurt, granola, mixed berries, and honey.
2. Repeat the layers as desired.

Vegetable Omelette

Ingredients:

- 2 egg whites

- 1/4 cup diced bell peppers
- 1/4 cup diced tomatoes
- 1/4 cup diced spinach
- Salt and pepper to taste

Instructions:

1. Whisk egg whites and season with salt and pepper.
2. Pour into a hot, non-stick pan and add diced vegetables.
3. Cook until the omelette is set, then fold in half.

Apple Cinnamon Quinoa

Ingredients:

- 1/2 cup cooked quinoa
- 1/2 apple, diced
- 1/4 teaspoon cinnamon
- 1 tablespoon chopped nuts

Instructions:

1. In a bowl, combine cooked quinoa, diced apple, and cinnamon.
2. Top with chopped nuts for added crunch and flavor.

Smoothie Bowl

Ingredients:

- 1/2 cup low-sodium yogurt
- 1/2 cup mixed berries
- 1/4 cup granola
- 1 tablespoon honey

Instructions:

1. Blend yogurt and mixed berries until smooth.
2. Pour the smoothie into a bowl, and top with granola and a drizzle of honey.

Low-Sodium Breakfast Burrito

Ingredients:

- 2 egg whites
- 1/4 cup diced tomatoes
- 1/4 cup diced bell peppers
- 1/4 cup diced onions
- Whole-grain tortilla

Instructions:

1. Scramble the egg whites and cook in a non-stick pan.
2. Place the cooked egg whites, diced vegetables, and a pinch of salt into a whole-grain tortilla.
3. Fold the tortilla and enjoy.

Cottage Cheese and Fruit

Ingredients:

*   1/2 cup low-sodium cottage cheese
*   1/2 cup mixed fruit (e.g., peaches, pineapple)

Instructions:

1. Serve a scoop of low-sodium cottage cheese in a bowl.
2. Top with mixed fruit for a refreshing and protein-rich breakfast.

Breakfast Muffins

Ingredients:

*   2 whole-grain muffins
*   2 tablespoons almond butter

- Sliced banana and strawberries

Instructions:

1. Spread almond butter on whole-grain muffins.
2. Top with sliced banana and strawberries for a delightful twist.

Avocado Toast

Ingredients:

- 1 slice of whole-grain bread
- 1/2 ripe avocado
- Sliced cherry tomatoes
- A pinch of salt and pepper

Instructions:

1. Toast the whole-grain bread.
2. Spread ripe avocado on the toast, then add sliced cherry tomatoes.
3. Season with a pinch of salt and pepper.

Rice Pudding

Ingredients:

- 1/2 cup cooked rice
- 1/2 cup low-sodium milk
- 1/4 teaspoon vanilla extract
- 1/4 teaspoon ground cinnamon

Instructions:

1. In a saucepan, combine cooked rice, low-sodium milk, vanilla extract, and ground cinnamon.
2. Cook, stirring occasionally, until the mixture thickens and is heated through.

Breakfast Quesadilla

Ingredients:

- 2 egg whites
- 1/4 cup diced bell peppers
- 1/4 cup diced onions
- Low-sodium cheese
- Whole-grain tortilla

Instructions:

1. Scramble the egg whites and cook in a non-stick pan.

2. Place the cooked egg whites, diced vegetables, and a sprinkle of low-sodium cheese inside a whole-grain tortilla.

3. Fold the tortilla and cook until the cheese melts.

Breakfast Casserole

Ingredients:

- 2 egg whites
- 1/2 cup diced vegetables (bell peppers, onions, spinach)
- 2 tablespoons low-sodium cheese

Instructions:

1. Whisk the egg whites and mix in diced vegetables.

2. Pour the mixture into a baking dish, top with low-sodium cheese, and bake until set.

Sweet Potato Hash

Ingredients:

- 1/2 cup diced sweet potatoes
- 1/4 cup diced onions
- 1/4 cup diced bell peppers
- Olive oil for cooking

Instructions:

1. Sauté diced sweet potatoes, onions, and bell peppers in a skillet with a touch of olive oil until tender and lightly browned.

Blueberry Waffles

Ingredients:

- Whole-grain waffles
- 1/2 cup fresh blueberries
- A drizzle of honey

Instructions:

1. Toast whole-grain waffles until crisp.
2. Top with fresh blueberries and a drizzle of honey.

Tofu Scramble

Ingredients:

- 1/2 cup crumbled tofu
- 1/4 cup diced tomatoes
- 1/4 cup diced onions
- 1/4 cup diced bell peppers
- A pinch of turmeric and black salt

Instructions:

1. Sauté crumbled tofu with diced vegetables, turmeric, and black salt until heated through.

Pumpkin Spice Porridge

Ingredients:

- 1/2 cup cooked brown rice
- 1/4 cup pumpkin puree
- 1/4 teaspoon pumpkin spice
- 1 tablespoon chopped nuts

Instructions:

1. Mix cooked brown rice with pumpkin puree and pumpkin spice.
2. Top with chopped nuts for added flavor and texture.

Chapter 3: Lunch Recipes

In Chapter 3, you'll find a delightful array of lunch recipes that are not only delicious but also suitable for your dialysis diet. These recipes are thoughtfully crafted to provide both flavor and nutrition to make your midday meal enjoyable. Let's explore these appetizing lunch options:

Chicken and Vegetable Stir-Fry

Ingredients:

- 1 boneless, skinless chicken breast, sliced
- 1 cup broccoli florets
- 1 bell pepper, thinly sliced
- 1/4 cup low-sodium stir-fry sauce
- 1 tablespoon vegetable oil
- Salt and pepper to taste

Instructions:

1. Heat vegetable oil in a pan over medium-high heat.
2. Add chicken and stir-fry until cooked through.

3. Add broccoli and bell pepper, stir-fry for a few minutes.

4. Pour in stir-fry sauce and cook until heated through.

5. Season with salt and pepper. Serve hot.

Tuna Salad with Avocado

Ingredients:

- 1 can of low-sodium tuna, drained
- 1 ripe avocado, diced
- 1/4 cup red onion, finely chopped
- 2 tablespoons lemon juice
- Salt and pepper to taste
- Fresh parsley for garnish

Instructions:

1. In a bowl, combine tuna, avocado, and red onion.

2. Drizzle with lemon juice and mix gently.

3. Season with salt and pepper.

4. Garnish with fresh parsley. Enjoy!

Spinach and Feta Stuffed Chicken

Ingredients:

- 2 boneless, skinless chicken breasts
- 1 cup fresh spinach leaves
- 1/4 cup crumbled feta cheese
- 1 tablespoon olive oil
- Salt and pepper to taste

Instructions:

1. Preheat the oven to 375°F (190°C).
2. Cut a pocket in each chicken breast.
3. Stuff each chicken breast with spinach and feta.
4. Brush with olive oil and season with salt and pepper.
5. Bake for 25-30 minutes or until chicken is cooked through.

Quinoa Salad with Roasted Vegetables

Ingredients:

- 1 cup cooked quinoa

- 1 cup mixed roasted vegetables (bell peppers, zucchini, carrots, etc.)
- 1/4 cup crumbled feta cheese
- 2 tablespoons balsamic vinaigrette
- Fresh basil leaves for garnish

Instructions:

1. In a bowl, combine cooked quinoa, roasted vegetables, and feta.
2. Drizzle with balsamic vinaigrette and toss gently.
3. Garnish with fresh basil leaves. Serve as a refreshing salad.

Mediterranean Chicken Wrap

Ingredients:

- 1 whole-grain tortilla
- 1 grilled chicken breast, sliced
- 1/4 cup hummus
- Sliced cucumbers, tomatoes, and red onions
- Fresh parsley for garnish

Instructions:

1. Lay out the tortilla.
2. Spread a layer of hummus in the center.
3. Add grilled chicken, cucumbers, tomatoes, and red onions.
4. Garnish with fresh parsley.
5. Wrap it up and enjoy this Mediterranean delight.

Shrimp and Asparagus Salad

Ingredients:

- 1 cup cooked shrimp
- Steamed asparagus spears
- Mixed greens
- Cherry tomatoes
- Balsamic vinaigrette
- Lemon wedges

Instructions:

1. Arrange mixed greens on a plate.
2. Top with cooked shrimp, steamed asparagus, and cherry tomatoes.
3. Drizzle with balsamic vinaigrette.

4. Serve with lemon wedges for extra zest.

Turkey and Cranberry Sandwich

Ingredients:

- 2 slices of whole-grain bread
- Sliced roasted turkey breast
- Cranberry sauce
- Spinach leaves
- Low-sodium mayonnaise

Instructions:

1. Spread a thin layer of mayonnaise on one slice of bread.
2. Layer turkey, cranberry sauce, and spinach leaves.
3. Top with the other slice of bread.
4. Slice in half and savor the turkey-cranberry combination.

Grilled Portobello Mushroom Burger

Ingredients:

- 2 large Portobello mushrooms

- Balsamic vinegar

- Olive oil

- Grilled bell pepper slices

- Whole-grain burger buns

Instructions:

1. Mix balsamic vinegar and olive oil to create a marinade.

2. Brush the mushrooms with the marinade.

3. Grill the mushrooms and bell pepper slices.

4. Place the grilled vegetables in a bun for a delicious burger.

Lentil Soup

Ingredients:

- 1 cup green or brown lentils

- Chopped carrots, celery, and onions

- Low-sodium vegetable broth

- Herbs and spices (such as thyme and bay leaves)

Instructions:

1. Combine lentils, vegetables, and broth in a pot.

2. Add herbs and spices.

3. Simmer until lentils are tender and vegetables are cooked.

4. Enjoy a hearty bowl of lentil soup.

Tofu and Broccoli Stir-Fry

Ingredients:

- Firm tofu, cubed
- Broccoli florets
- Low-sodium stir-fry sauce
- Sliced green onions
- Sesame seeds

Instructions:

1. In a pan, stir-fry tofu until it begins to brown.

2. Add broccoli, green onions, and stir-fry sauce.

3. Cook until broccoli is tender.

4. Garnish with sesame seeds and serve with brown rice.

Chicken Noodle Soup

Ingredients:

- 1 cup cooked chicken, shredded
- Low-sodium chicken broth
- Cooked whole-wheat noodles
- Sliced carrots and celery
- Fresh parsley

Instructions:

1. Combine chicken, broth, and vegetables in a pot.
2. Simmer until vegetables are tender.
3. Add cooked noodles.
4. Garnish with fresh parsley and enjoy comforting soup.

Caprese Salad

Ingredients:

- Fresh tomatoes, sliced
- Fresh mozzarella cheese, sliced
- Fresh basil leaves
- Balsamic glaze

- Olive oil

Instructions:

1. Arrange tomato and mozzarella slices on a plate.
2. Tuck in fresh basil leaves.
3. Drizzle with balsamic glaze and olive oil.
4. Savor this classic Italian salad.

Salmon and Brown Rice

Ingredients:

- Baked or grilled salmon fillet
- Cooked brown rice
- Steamed broccoli
- Lemon wedges
- Dill for garnish

Instructions:

1. Place salmon on a bed of brown rice.
2. Serve with steamed broccoli.
3. Garnish with lemon wedges and dill.
4. Enjoy a nutritious and flavorful meal.

Egg Salad Lettuce Wraps

Ingredients:

- Hard-boiled eggs, chopped
- Greek yogurt
- Diced celery and red onion
- Lettuce leaves
- Dill for seasoning

Instructions:

1. Mix chopped eggs, Greek yogurt, celery, and red onion.
2. Season with dill.
3. Spoon the mixture into lettuce leaves.
4. Roll up and savor these refreshing lettuce wraps.

Black Bean and Corn Salad

Ingredients:

- Black beans
- Corn kernels
- Chopped bell peppers and red onions
- Cilantro

- Lime juice

- Cumin and chili powder

Instructions:

1. Combine black beans, corn, bell peppers, and red onions.

2. Add cilantro, lime juice, cumin, and chili powder.

3. Toss well for a zesty and healthy salad.

Minestrone Soup

Ingredients:

- Low-sodium vegetable broth

- Chopped carrots, celery, and zucchini

- Cooked kidney beans

- Whole-wheat pasta

- Fresh basil

Instructions:

1. Bring broth, vegetables, and beans to a simmer.

2. Add cooked pasta and fresh basil.

3. Serve this hearty Italian soup.

Hummus and Veggie Wrap

Ingredients:

- Whole-grain tortilla
- Hummus
- Sliced cucumber, red bell pepper, and carrots
- Spinach leaves

Instructions:

1. Spread hummus on the tortilla.
2. Add sliced vegetables and spinach leaves.
3. Roll up and enjoy a delightful wrap.

Stuffed Bell Peppers

Ingredients:

- Bell peppers, halved and seeded
- Ground turkey or lean beef
- Cooked quinoa
- Diced tomatoes
- Italian seasoning
- Shredded low-fat cheese

Instructions:

1. Brown meat, add cooked quinoa, tomatoes, and seasoning.

2. Stuff bell pepper halves with the mixture.

3. Top with cheese and bake until peppers are tender.

Chapter 4: Dinner Recipes

In this chapter, you'll discover a delightful collection of dinner recipes tailored for a Dialysis Diet. These recipes are not only nutritious but also packed with flavor to make your dinners enjoyable. Remember, maintaining a balanced diet is crucial for those on dialysis, and these recipes are designed with that in mind. Let's dive into a world of delicious and kidney-friendly dinners:

Baked Salmon with Dill

Ingredients:

- 4 salmon fillets
- 1 tablespoon olive oil
- 1 teaspoon dried dill
- Salt and pepper to taste
- 2 lemons, sliced

Instructions:

1. Preheat your oven to 375°F (190°C).
2. Place salmon fillets on a baking sheet.

3. Drizzle with olive oil and sprinkle with dill, salt, and pepper.

4. Lay lemon slices over the fillets.

5. Bake for 15-20 minutes, or until the salmon flakes easily with a fork.

Lemon Herb Grilled Chicken

Ingredients:

- 4 boneless, skinless chicken breasts
- Zest and juice of 1 lemon
- 2 cloves garlic, minced
- 1 tablespoon fresh thyme, chopped
- Salt and pepper to taste

Instructions:

1. In a bowl, mix lemon zest, lemon juice, minced garlic, and thyme.

2. Season chicken breasts with salt and pepper, then brush with the lemon herb mixture.

3. Grill the chicken until cooked through, approximately 6-8 minutes per side.

Vegetable and Lentil Curry

Ingredients:

- 1 cup red lentils
- 2 cups water
- 2 tablespoons olive oil
- 1 onion, chopped
- 2 cloves garlic, minced
- 1 tablespoon curry powder
- 2 cups mixed vegetables (e.g., bell peppers, zucchini, carrots)
- 1 can diced tomatoes
- Salt and pepper to taste

Instructions:

1. Rinse lentils and cook them in 2 cups of water until tender.
2. In a separate pot, sauté onions and garlic in olive oil.
3. Stir in curry powder and cook briefly.
4. Add mixed vegetables and diced tomatoes, then simmer until vegetables are tender.
5. Mix in cooked lentils, season with salt and pepper, and let it simmer for a few more minutes.

Beef and Vegetable Skewers

Ingredients:

- 1 pound lean beef, cut into cubes
- 1 red bell pepper, cut into chunks
- 1 yellow bell pepper, cut into chunks
- 1 red onion, cut into chunks
- 1 zucchini, sliced
- Marinade: 2 tablespoons olive oil, 2 cloves garlic (minced), 1 teaspoon dried oregano, salt, and pepper

Instructions:

1. Combine the marinade ingredients in a bowl.
2. Thread the beef and vegetables onto skewers.
3. Brush with the marinade and grill until the beef is cooked to your preference.

Spaghetti Squash with Pesto

Ingredients:

- 1 spaghetti squash
- 2 cups fresh basil leaves
- 1/2 cup grated Parmesan cheese

- 1/2 cup pine nuts

- 2 cloves garlic

- 1/4 cup olive oil

- Salt and pepper to taste

Instructions:

1. Cut the spaghetti squash in half, remove seeds, and roast in the oven until tender.

2. In a food processor, combine basil, Parmesan, pine nuts, garlic, olive oil, salt, and pepper to make the pesto sauce.

3. Scrape the spaghetti squash with a fork to create "noodles" and toss with the pesto.

Tofu and Broccoli in Garlic Sauce

Ingredients:

- 1 block of tofu, cubed

- 2 cups broccoli florets

- Sauce: 1/4 cup low-sodium soy sauce, 1 tablespoon minced garlic, 1 tablespoon honey, 1 teaspoon ginger (minced)

Instructions:

1. In a pan, stir-fry tofu until golden brown. Remove and set aside.
2. Stir-fry broccoli until tender.
3. In a small bowl, whisk together the sauce ingredients.
4. Add tofu back to the pan, pour the sauce over the tofu and broccoli, and cook for a few minutes until heated through.

Roast Turkey with Gravy

Ingredients:

- 1 turkey breast (skinless)
- 1 teaspoon olive oil
- 1 teaspoon dried thyme
- Salt and pepper to taste

Instructions:

1. Preheat your oven to 350°F (175°C).
2. Rub the turkey breast with olive oil, thyme, salt, and pepper.
3. Roast the turkey until it reaches an internal temperature of 165°F (74°C), usually about 1 hour.

Cod with Lemon Butter

Ingredients:

- 4 cod fillets
- 2 tablespoons unsalted butter
- Juice of 1 lemon
- 1 teaspoon fresh parsley, chopped
- Salt and pepper to taste

Instructions:

1. In a pan, melt butter and add lemon juice and parsley.
2. Season cod fillets with salt and pepper.
3. Cook the cod in the lemon butter sauce until it flakes easily.

Chickpea and Spinach Stew

Ingredients:

- 2 cans chickpeas, drained and rinsed
- 2 cups fresh spinach
- 1 onion, chopped
- 2 cloves garlic, minced
- 1 teaspoon ground cumin

- 1/2 teaspoon paprika

- Salt and pepper to taste

Instructions:

1. Sauté onions and garlic in a pot until softened.

2. Add chickpeas, cumin, paprika, and cook for a few minutes.

3. Stir in fresh spinach and cook until wilted.

Pork Tenderloin with Apples

Ingredients:

- 1 pork tenderloin

- 2 apples, sliced

- 1 tablespoon olive oil

- 1 teaspoon dried rosemary

- Salt and pepper to taste

Instructions:

1. Preheat your oven to 375°F (190°C).

2. Season the pork with rosemary, salt, and pepper.

3. In a pan, sear the pork until browned on all sides.

4. Place apples in the same pan and transfer to the oven. Roast until the pork is cooked through and the apples are tender.

Baked Eggplant Parmesan

Ingredients:

- 2 large eggplants, sliced
- 2 cups marinara sauce
- 1 cup shredded mozzarella cheese
- 1/2 cup grated Parmesan cheese
- Fresh basil leaves for garnish
- Salt and pepper to taste

Instructions:

1. Preheat your oven to 375°F (190°C).
2. Dip eggplant slices in marinara sauce and arrange in a baking dish.
3. Sprinkle with mozzarella and Parmesan cheese.
4. Bake until the cheese is bubbly and golden.
5. Garnish with fresh basil leaves.

Salsa Chicken

Ingredients:

- 4 boneless, skinless chicken breasts
- 1 cup salsa
- 1 cup shredded cheddar cheese
- Salt and pepper to taste

Instructions:

1. Preheat your oven to 375°F (190°C).
2. Season chicken breasts with salt and pepper.
3. Pour salsa over chicken and top with cheddar cheese.
4. Bake until the chicken is cooked through and the cheese is melted and bubbly.

Teriyaki Beef Stir-Fry

Ingredients:

- 1 pound lean beef, sliced
- 1 cup broccoli florets
- 1 cup sliced bell peppers
- 1 cup snap peas
- 1/2 cup low-sodium teriyaki sauce

- 1 tablespoon vegetable oil

- Sesame seeds for garnish

Instructions:

1. In a wok or large skillet, heat the vegetable oil.

2. Stir-fry beef until browned, then set it aside.

3. In the same pan, stir-fry vegetables until tender-crisp.

4. Return beef to the pan and add teriyaki sauce.

5. Cook briefly, then garnish with sesame seeds.

Ratatouille

Ingredients:

- 2 small zucchinis, sliced

- 1 eggplant, cubed

- 2 red bell peppers, sliced

- 2 tomatoes, diced

- 1 onion, chopped

- 2 cloves garlic, minced

- 1/4 cup olive oil

- 1 teaspoon dried thyme

- Salt and pepper to taste

Instructions:

1. In a large pot, heat olive oil and sauté onions and garlic.

2. Layer the vegetables in the pot, seasoning each layer with thyme, salt, and pepper.

3. Cover and simmer until the vegetables are tender.

BBQ Pulled Chicken

Ingredients:

- 4 boneless, skinless chicken breasts
- 1 cup low-sodium barbecue sauce
- 1/4 cup apple cider vinegar
- 1/4 cup brown sugar
- 1/2 teaspoon garlic powder
- 1/2 teaspoon onion powder

Instructions:

1. Place chicken breasts in a slow cooker.

2. In a bowl, mix barbecue sauce, vinegar, brown sugar, garlic powder, and onion powder.

3. Pour the sauce over the chicken.

4. Cook on low for 6-7 hours or until chicken is easily shredded.

Shrimp Scampi

Ingredients:

- 1 pound large shrimp, peeled and deveined
- 4 cloves garlic, minced
- 1/4 cup white wine
- 1/4 cup low-sodium chicken broth
- 2 tablespoons fresh lemon juice
- 2 tablespoons fresh parsley, chopped
- 2 tablespoons butter
- Salt and pepper to taste

Instructions:

1. In a pan, melt butter and sauté garlic until fragrant.
2. Add shrimp and cook until pink, then remove and set aside.
3. In the same pan, add white wine, chicken broth, lemon juice, and parsley.
4. Simmer until reduced, then pour the sauce over the shrimp.

Vegetable Lasagna

Ingredients:

- 12 lasagna noodles (cooked)
- 3 cups low-fat ricotta cheese
- 2 cups shredded mozzarella cheese
- 2 cups marinara sauce
- 2 cups mixed vegetables (e.g., spinach, zucchini, mushrooms)
- Salt and pepper to taste

Instructions:

1. Preheat your oven to 375°F (190°C).
2. In a baking dish, layer cooked lasagna noodles, ricotta cheese, vegetables, mozzarella, and marinara sauce.
3. Repeat the layers.
4. Bake until the lasagna is hot and bubbly.

Beef and Rice Stuffed Peppers

Ingredients:

- 4 bell peppers

- 1 pound lean ground beef
- 1 cup cooked rice
- 1 can diced tomatoes
- 1 teaspoon dried oregano
- Salt and pepper to taste

Instructions:

1. Preheat your oven to 375°F (190°C).
2. Cut the tops off the bell peppers and remove seeds.
3. In a bowl, mix beef, cooked rice, diced tomatoes, oregano, salt, and pepper.
4. Stuff the peppers with the mixture and bake until the peppers are tender.

Chapter 5: Snacks and Appetizers

When it comes to snacks and appetizers for your dialysis diet, you don't have to compromise on flavor or variety. In this chapter, we've curated delightful options that not only taste fantastic but are also kidney-friendly. These snacks and appetizers are perfect for satisfying your cravings and keeping your diet on track.

Cucumber Slices with Hummus

Ingredients:

- Fresh cucumbers, thinly sliced
- Low-sodium hummus

Instructions:

1. Slice the cucumbers into thin rounds.
2. Serve them with a side of low-sodium hummus for dipping.

Roasted Red Pepper Dip

Ingredients:

- Roasted red peppers (you can roast them at home or use jarred)
- Greek yogurt
- Garlic, minced
- Olive oil
- Lemon juice
- Salt and pepper to taste

Instructions:

1. Blend roasted red peppers, Greek yogurt, minced garlic, olive oil, lemon juice, salt, and pepper until smooth.
2. Serve with your favorite low-sodium crackers or vegetable sticks.

Greek Salad Skewers

Ingredients:

- Cherry tomatoes
- Cucumber, cut into chunks

- Red onion, cut into small pieces
- Feta cheese, cubed
- Kalamata olives
- Fresh basil leaves
- Balsamic glaze (optional)

Instructions:

1. Thread cherry tomatoes, cucumber, red onion, feta cheese, Kalamata olives, and basil leaves onto skewers.
2. Drizzle with balsamic glaze if desired.

Mixed Nuts

Ingredients:

- Assorted unsalted mixed nuts (almonds, walnuts, cashews)

Instructions:

1. Simply mix your favorite unsalted nuts and enjoy as a protein-packed snack.

Deviled Eggs

Ingredients:

- Hard-boiled eggs
- Low-fat mayonnaise
- Dijon mustard
- Paprika
- Salt and pepper

Instructions:

1. Cut hard-boiled eggs in half, remove yolks, and mash them.
2. Mix yolks with low-fat mayonnaise, Dijon mustard, paprika, salt, and pepper.
3. Fill egg whites with the yolk mixture.

Guacamole with Veggie Sticks

Ingredients:

- Ripe avocados
- Lime juice
- Red onion, finely chopped
- Tomatoes, diced

- Cilantro, chopped
- Salt and pepper
- Assorted vegetable sticks (carrots, bell peppers, cucumber)

Instructions:

1. Mash avocados and mix with lime juice, red onion, tomatoes, cilantro, salt, and pepper.
2. Serve with assorted vegetable sticks for dipping.

Rice Cakes with Peanut Butter

Ingredients:

- Low-sodium rice cakes
- Natural peanut butter (unsalted)

Instructions:

1. Spread a thin layer of natural peanut butter on low-sodium rice cakes for a crunchy, satisfying snack.

Zucchini Fritters

Ingredients:

- Grated zucchini
- Eggs
- Chopped scallions
- Whole wheat flour
- Salt and pepper
- Olive oil for cooking

Instructions:

1. Combine grated zucchini, eggs, chopped scallions, whole wheat flour, salt, and pepper.
2. Heat olive oil in a pan, spoon the mixture onto the pan, and cook until golden brown on both sides.

Fruit Kabobs

Ingredients:

- Assorted fruits (e.g., melon, grapes, berries)
- Wooden skewers

Instructions:

1. Thread bite-sized fruit pieces onto wooden skewers to create colorful and refreshing fruit kabobs.

Caprese Skewers

Ingredients:

- Cherry tomatoes
- Fresh mozzarella balls
- Fresh basil leaves
- Balsamic glaze (optional)

Instructions:

1. Thread cherry tomatoes, fresh mozzarella balls, and basil leaves onto skewers.
2. Drizzle with balsamic glaze for extra flavor.

Baked Sweet Potato Fries

Ingredients:

- Sweet potatoes, cut into fries
- Olive oil
- Paprika

- Salt and pepper

Instructions:

1. Toss sweet potato fries with olive oil, paprika, salt, and pepper.
2. Bake in the oven until crispy and golden brown.

Spinach and Artichoke Dip

Ingredients:

- Spinach, chopped
- Artichoke hearts, chopped
- Low-fat cream cheese
- Greek yogurt
- Garlic, minced
- Parmesan cheese
- Salt and pepper

Instructions:

1. Mix chopped spinach, artichoke hearts, low-fat cream cheese, Greek yogurt, minced garlic, Parmesan cheese, salt, and pepper.
2. Warm in the oven and serve with veggie sticks.

Cottage Cheese with Pineapple

Ingredients:

- Low-fat cottage cheese
- Pineapple chunks

Instructions:

1. Top low-fat cottage cheese with pineapple chunks for a sweet and savory snack.

Edamame

Ingredients:

- Edamame beans (steamed or boiled)
- Sea salt

Instructions:

1. Sprinkle edamame beans with sea salt and enjoy as a protein-rich snack.

Mini Quiches

Ingredients:

- Whole wheat mini quiche shells

- Eggs
- Low-fat milk
- Spinach, chopped
- Cheddar cheese, grated
- Salt and pepper

Instructions:

1. Whisk eggs and low-fat milk, then add chopped spinach, grated cheddar cheese, salt, and pepper.
2. Pour the mixture into mini quiche shells and bake until set.

Baked Pita Chips with Salsa

Ingredients:

- Whole wheat pita bread
- Olive oil
- Paprika
- Salt
- Tomato salsa

Instructions:

1. Cut pita bread into triangles, brush with olive oil, sprinkle with paprika and salt.

2. Bake until crisp and serve with tomato salsa.

Tzatziki and Pita Bread

Ingredients:

- Greek yogurt
- Cucumber, grated
- Garlic, minced
- Fresh dill, chopped
- Lemon juice
- Whole wheat pita bread

Instructions:

1. Mix Greek yogurt, grated cucumber, minced garlic, chopped dill, and lemon juice to create tzatziki.

2. Serve with whole wheat pita bread.

Veggie Spring Rolls

Ingredients:

- Rice paper wrappers
- Mixed vegetables (carrots, cucumber, bell peppers)
- Fresh herbs (mint, cilantro)
- Dipping sauce (low-sodium soy sauce with lime and ginger)

Instructions:

1. Soak rice paper wrappers in warm water until soft.
2. Fill with mixed vegetables and fresh herbs, then roll them up.
3. Serve with the dipping sauce.

Chapter 6: Desserts

In this chapter, we will explore a variety of sweet treats that not only satisfy your cravings but also adhere to the dietary restrictions necessary for a healthier life. From refreshing fruit sorbets to creamy pudding alternatives, we've got your dessert cravings covered.

Berry Sorbet

Ingredients:

- 2 cups mixed berries (strawberries, blueberries, raspberries)
- 1/4 cup water
- 1/4 cup sugar substitute
- 1 tablespoon lemon juice

Instructions:

1. In a blender, combine the mixed berries and water. Blend until smooth.
2. Add the sugar substitute and lemon juice, and blend again until well combined.

3. Pour the mixture into a shallow dish and freeze for 4-6 hours.

4. Serve your refreshing berry sorbet and enjoy.

Poached Pears

Ingredients:

- 2 ripe pears, peeled and cored
- 2 cups water
- 1/4 cup sugar substitute
- 1 cinnamon stick
- 1 teaspoon lemon zest

Instructions:

1. In a pot, combine water, sugar substitute, cinnamon stick, and lemon zest.

2. Bring the mixture to a simmer and add the pears.

3. Simmer gently for about 20-25 minutes until the pears are tender but not mushy.

4. Remove pears from the poaching liquid and let them cool.

5. Serve the poached pears with a drizzle of the poaching liquid.

Applesauce with Cinnamon

Ingredients:

- 2 cups unsweetened applesauce
- 1/2 teaspoon ground cinnamon
- 1 tablespoon sugar substitute

Instructions:

1. In a bowl, mix the unsweetened applesauce with ground cinnamon and sugar substitute.
2. Stir until the ingredients are well combined.
3. Chill in the refrigerator for at least 30 minutes.
4. Sprinkle a little extra cinnamon on top before serving.

Chia Seed Pudding

Ingredients:

- 1/4 cup chia seeds
- 1 cup unsweetened almond milk
- 1/2 teaspoon vanilla extract
- 1 tablespoon sugar substitute

Instructions:

1. In a jar, combine chia seeds, almond milk, vanilla extract, and sugar substitute.

2. Stir well and refrigerate for at least 2 hours, or overnight.

3. Before serving, give it a good stir and add your favorite berries on top.

Angel Food Cake with Berries

Ingredients:

- 1 slice of angel food cake
- 1/4 cup mixed berries (strawberries, blueberries, raspberries)
- 1 tablespoon sugar-free whipped topping

Instructions:

1. Place a slice of angel food cake on a dessert plate.

2. Top it with mixed berries.

3. Add a dollop of sugar-free whipped topping.

4. Savor this guilt-free dessert.

Rice Pudding

Ingredients:

- 1/2 cup cooked white rice
- 1 cup unsweetened almond milk
- 1/2 teaspoon vanilla extract
- 1/4 teaspoon ground cinnamon
- 1 tablespoon sugar substitute

Instructions:

1. In a saucepan, combine cooked rice, almond milk, vanilla extract, ground cinnamon, and sugar substitute.
2. Cook on low heat, stirring occasionally, until the mixture thickens (about 15-20 minutes).
3. Remove from heat and let it cool before serving.

Pumpkin Pie Smoothie

Ingredients:

- 1/2 cup canned pumpkin puree
- 1/2 cup unsweetened almond milk
- 1/2 teaspoon pumpkin pie spice

- 1 tablespoon sugar substitute
- Ice cubes

Instructions:

1. In a blender, combine pumpkin puree, almond milk, pumpkin pie spice, and sugar substitute.
2. Add ice cubes and blend until smooth.
3. Pour into a glass and enjoy the taste of fall in a refreshing smoothie.

Baked Apples

Ingredients:

- 2 apples, cored
- 1/4 cup sugar substitute
- 1/2 teaspoon ground cinnamon
- 1 tablespoon chopped nuts (optional)

Instructions:

1. Preheat your oven to 350°F (175°C).
2. In a small bowl, mix sugar substitute and ground cinnamon.
3. Fill the cored apples with the cinnamon mixture.

4. Place the apples in a baking dish and bake for 30-40 minutes, until tender.

5. If desired, sprinkle chopped nuts on top before serving.

Greek Yogurt with Honey

Ingredients:

- 1/2 cup low-fat Greek yogurt
- 1 tablespoon honey
- Fresh berries for topping

Instructions:

1. In a bowl, combine Greek yogurt and honey.
2. Top with fresh berries for a burst of flavor.
3. Enjoy this simple and nutritious dessert.

Chocolate Avocado Mousse

Ingredients:

- 1 ripe avocado
- 2 tablespoons unsweetened cocoa powder
- 1 tablespoon sugar substitute

- 1/2 teaspoon vanilla extract

Instructions:

1. In a blender, combine the avocado, cocoa powder, sugar substitute, and vanilla extract.
2. Blend until smooth and creamy.
3. Chill in the refrigerator before serving.

Banana Ice Cream

Ingredients:

- 2 ripe bananas, sliced and frozen
- 1/2 teaspoon vanilla extract
- 1 tablespoon sugar substitute

Instructions:

1. Place the frozen banana slices in a blender.
2. Add vanilla extract and sugar substitute.
3. Blend until the mixture has a creamy, ice cream-like texture.
4. Serve immediately for a refreshing treat.

Coconut Rice Pudding

Ingredients:

- 1/2 cup cooked rice
- 1/2 cup light coconut milk
- 1 tablespoon sugar substitute
- 1/4 teaspoon vanilla extract

Instructions:

1. In a saucepan, combine cooked rice, coconut milk, sugar substitute, and vanilla extract.
2. Cook on low heat, stirring until the mixture thickens (about 15-20 minutes).
3. Remove from heat and let it cool before serving.

Fruit Salad

Ingredients:

- A variety of fresh, diced fruits (e.g., melon, berries, pineapple, grapes)
- A drizzle of fresh lemon juice
- Optional: a sprinkle of chopped mint leaves

Instructions:

1. In a bowl, combine the diced fruits.

2. Drizzle with fresh lemon juice to enhance the flavors.

3. If desired, add a sprinkle of chopped mint leaves for extra freshness.

Frozen Yogurt Bites

Ingredients:

- Low-fat yogurt (flavor of your choice)
- Fresh berries or fruit pieces

Instructions:

1. Drop spoonfuls of yogurt onto a baking sheet.

2. Top each spoonful with fresh berries or fruit pieces.

3. Freeze for at least 2 hours.

4. Enjoy these bite-sized, frozen delights.

Peach Cobbler

Ingredients:

- 2 cups sliced canned peaches (in juice, not syrup)
- 1/2 cup rolled oats

- 1/4 cup almond meal
- 1/2 teaspoon cinnamon
- 1 tablespoon sugar substitute

Instructions:

1. Preheat your oven to 350°F (175°C).
2. In a baking dish, combine sliced peaches with a little juice, oats, almond meal, cinnamon, and sugar substitute.
3. Bake for 25-30 minutes, or until the topping is golden brown.
4. Serve warm.

Lemon Sorbet

Ingredients:

- 1 cup freshly squeezed lemon juice
- 1/2 cup water
- 1/4 cup sugar substitute
- Zest from one lemon

Instructions:

1. In a bowl, mix lemon juice, water, sugar substitute, and lemon zest.

2. Pour the mixture into an ice cream maker and churn according to the manufacturer's instructions.

3. Enjoy your homemade lemon sorbet.

Carrot Cake Bites

Ingredients:

- 1 cup grated carrots
- 1/2 cup unsweetened shredded coconut
- 1/4 cup chopped nuts (e.g., walnuts or almonds)
- 1/4 cup rolled oats
- 1 tablespoon sugar substitute
- 1/2 teaspoon ground cinnamon

Instructions:

1. In a bowl, combine grated carrots, shredded coconut, chopped nuts, oats, sugar substitute, and ground cinnamon.

2. Form the mixture into small bites and refrigerate for about an hour.

3. Enjoy these nutritious and satisfying carrot cake
   bites.

Almond Butter Cookies

Ingredients:

- 1 cup almond butter
- 1/4 cup sugar substitute
- 1 egg
- 1/2 teaspoon vanilla extract

Instructions:

1. Preheat your oven to 350°F (175°C).
2. In a bowl, combine almond butter, sugar substitute, egg, and vanilla extract.
3. Form small cookie rounds and place them on a baking sheet.
4. Bake for 10-12 minutes or until the edges are golden.
5. Let them cool before serving.

CONCLUSION

In the final chapter of our journey through dialysis diet meal plans, we wrap up with a sense of achievement and hope for the future. This chapter isn't just an ending; it's a new beginning, a launchpad for you to continue your path to better health and well-being.

As you've discovered throughout this book, the dialysis diet isn't just about restrictions; it's about possibilities. It's about exploring new flavors, trying different ingredients, and reimagining your relationship with food. You've learned that even within the confines of dietary restrictions, there's room for creativity, deliciousness, and satisfaction.

This is the part where we express our gratitude for your commitment to your health. We acknowledge the challenges you face, the effort you've put in, and the courage you've shown. We're grateful for the opportunity to be a part of your path towards a healthier and more vibrant life.

As we close this book, remember that the journey doesn't stop here. Your adventure in discovering delicious, kidney-friendly recipes and maintaining a dialysis diet continues. Embrace it with the knowledge, confidence, and inspiration you've gained from this guide. Keep exploring, keep cooking, and keep savoring the flavors of a life well-lived.

Thank you for being a part of this culinary voyage. Your health and well-being are worth every effort, and we're confident that you have the tools and the spirit to make it a rewarding and delicious one.

www.ingramcontent.com/pod-product-compliance
Lightning Source LLC
Chambersburg PA
CBHW050832260726
48660CB00006B/2187